Transform Your Health with Digital Wellness

Leverage Wearable Devices, Mobile Apps, AI Coaches, and Data to Optimize Fitness, Nutrition, Sleep, Preventative Care and Mental Wellbeing

M.H. Marks

Table of Contents

Introduction

Welcome to a transformative journey that holds the key to unlocking not just a healthier you, but a future of boundless possibilities. In the hustle of our daily lives, we often dream of a time when health, wealth, and happiness converge seamlessly. What if I told you that this dream is not only within reach but can be realized through the power of digital wellness?

In the next few minutes, envision a life where every step you take, every bite you savor, and every rejuvenating night's sleep contribute not just to your physical well-being but propels you towards financial freedom. Picture a world where your pursuit of a healthier lifestyle aligns with unprecedented opportunities to earn online. The convergence of health and wealth is not a distant reality, it's a journey we're about to embark on together.

As you turn these pages, consider the landscape of possibilities that the digital era unfolds before you. The internet, a vast ecosystem of opportunities, has become the gateway to financial liberation. The fusion of wearable devices, mobile apps, AI coaches, and data holds the promise of not just transforming your health but also reshaping your financial future.

What does this book promise to deliver? Practical insights, actionable strategies, and a roadmap to not just improve your health but to leverage your pursuit of wellness into a powerful online presence. You'll learn how your journey towards a healthier lifestyle can be seamlessly woven into the fabric of a thriving online venture.

Feel the urgency, the pulse of this moment. The time is now. The opportunities are ripe, and the convergence of health and wealth is calling out to you. In the pages that follow, we'll explore not just the "how" but the "why" behind each step, anchoring your actions in a relatable and urgent context.

Are you ready to turn the page towards a life where your health is not just an investment in your well-being but a pathway to financial freedom? Let's dive into the first chapter, where the first steps await you, a journey that begins with the turn of a page and propels you into a world of possibilities. Your transformation starts now.

Chapter 1

Foundations of Digital Wellness

Understanding Wearable Devices

Welcome to the starting line of your journey into the world of digital wellness! In this chapter, we'll lay the groundwork for your understanding of two essential pillars, Wearable Devices and Mobile Apps for Health. Think of these as your trusty companions on the path to a healthier and wealthier you.

Understanding Wearable Devices

What Are Wearable Devices?
Imagine having a mini health assistant right on your wrist or clipped to your clothing. That's what a wearable device is, a smart gadget designed to monitor various aspects of your health and daily activities. These nifty tools can track your steps, measure your heart rate, monitor sleep patterns, and more.

Step-by-Step:

1. Pick Your Wearable: Choose a device that suits your lifestyle and preferences. Whether it's a fitness tracker, smartwatch, or a specialized health monitor, there's something for everyone.

2. Sync and Connect: Pair your wearable with your smartphone. Most devices come with user-friendly apps to make this process a breeze.

3. Set Your Goals: Define your health goals within the app. Whether it's hitting a step count or improving sleep quality, your wearable is your motivator.

Real-World Example:

Meet Sarah, a busy professional. By using her fitness tracker, she discovered she was consistently missing her daily step goal. This insight prompted her to take short walks during breaks, not only improving her health but also boosting her productivity.

Exploring Mobile Apps for Health

The Power of Health Apps

Your smartphone is more than just a communication tool, it's a gateway to a multitude of health apps designed to enhance your well-being. From nutrition trackers to workout guides, these apps put the control of your health in the palm of your hand.

Step-by-Step:

1. Research and Download: Explore app stores for apps that align with your health goals. Read reviews and choose those with user-friendly interfaces.

2. Set Personal Targets: Most apps allow you to set personalized goals. Whether it's weight loss, mindful eating, or meditation, define your objectives.

3. Consistent Tracking: Use the app regularly to track your progress. Many apps provide insights and tips based on your data.

Real-World Example:

John struggled with maintaining a balanced diet. He started using a nutrition app that not only tracked his meals but also provided healthy recipes and grocery lists. Over time, he not only improved his eating habits but also discovered a passion for cooking.

Recap and Moving Forward

Congratulations! You've now laid the groundwork for your digital wellness journey. You understand how wearable devices and health apps can be your allies in this adventure. Now, it's time to get hands-on.

Key Takeaways:
- Wearables are like personal health assistants, providing real-time data and motivation.
- Health apps turn your smartphone into a hub for wellness, offering tools for nutrition, exercise, and more.

Introduction to AI Coaches

Welcome to the next phase of your digital wellness journey! In this chapter, we'll delve into the fascinating realm of AI Coaches and the incredible power of harnessing data for optimizing your health. Picture having a virtual guide by your side, analyzing your habits and offering personalized insights to propel you towards your health and financial goals. Let's jump in!

Introduction to AI Coaches

What is an AI Coach?
Think of an AI Coach as your health guru powered by artificial intelligence. These digital mentors analyze vast amounts of data, learn about your habits, and tailor recommendations to fit your unique needs. It's like having a knowledgeable friend who knows exactly what you need to stay on track.

Getting Started:
1. Choose Your AI Coach: Explore available AI coaching platforms. Some focus on fitness, others on mental well-being, and some offer a holistic approach.

2. Personalize Your Profile: Input your health goals, preferences, and any relevant health data.

The more information you provide, the more accurate your AI Coach becomes.

3. Engage and Learn: Regularly interact with your AI Coach. Answer questions, share updates, and let the AI adapt to your evolving needs.

Harnessing Data for Health Optimization

The Power of Data in Wellness

Your journey towards better health involves more than just steps and sleep patterns. It's about understanding the nuances of your lifestyle, and that's where data comes into play. AI Coaches thrive on data, using it to provide targeted advice, identify trends, and empower you to make informed decisions.

Simple Steps:

1. Connect Your Devices: Ensure your wearables and health apps are synced with your AI Coach platform. This allows for comprehensive data analysis.

2. Regular Check-Ins: Make a habit of updating your AI Coach with relevant information. The more accurate the data, the more precise the recommendations.

3. Review and Adjust: Periodically review the insights provided by your AI Coach. Use this information to tweak your health goals and refine your strategies.

Recap and Moving Forward

You've now stepped into the world of AI Coaches and the profound impact of data in health optimization. As you embrace these digital guides, remember that the more you engage and share, the more customized and effective the advice becomes.

Key Takeaways:
- AI Coaches leverage artificial intelligence to provide personalized health guidance.
- Data is the backbone of effective health optimization, empowering AI Coaches to offer tailored insights.

Ready for the next adventure? In Chapter 2, we'll explore how wearable devices can supercharge your fitness journey. How do you envision AI Coaches enhancing your wellness routine? Share your thoughts in the comments below and let the digital conversation begin!

Chapter 2

Fitness Enhancement through Digital Tools

Fitness Tracking with Wearables

Welcome to the heart of your digital wellness journey, where fitness meets technology in an exhilarating dance of progress and achievement. In this chapter, we'll dive into the world of fitness tracking with wearables, unlocking the potential for a healthier, more active you.

Fitness Tracking with Wearables

The Wearable Revolution

Imagine having a personal fitness companion that goes beyond counting steps. Wearables are your dynamic sidekick, equipped with sensors that monitor everything from heart rate to sleep patterns. They're not just accessories; they're your partners in progress.

Getting Started:

1. Select Your Wearable: Choose a device that aligns with your fitness goals. Whether it's a sleek smartwatch or a dedicated fitness tracker, find the one that suits your style and needs.

2. Strap It On: Make your wearable a part of your daily routine. Wear it consistently to ensure accurate tracking of your movements, workouts, and overall activity.

3. Sync and Go: Connect your wearable to its accompanying app on your smartphone. This step is crucial for accessing detailed insights and personalized recommendations.

The Power of Real-Time Feedback

Your wearable is more than just a stylish accessory, it's a real-time feedback system. As you move, exercise, and rest, your device keeps you informed, motivated, and on the path to achieving your fitness aspirations.

Making Every Step Count

Setting and Achieving Goals

One of the magic elements of wearables is their ability to turn every step into a tangible goal. Whether it's reaching a daily step count or conquering a new running distance, your wearable transforms ordinary activities into milestones of achievement.

Simple Steps:

1. Define Your Goals: Set achievable yet challenging fitness goals. Your wearable can help you break them down into daily targets.

2. Celebrate Milestones: Revel in your successes, no matter how small. Wearables often reward you with badges or encouraging messages, turning your fitness journey into a game of accomplishment.

3. Adjust and Progress: As you hit your initial goals, adjust them to ensure a continuous challenge. Your wearable evolves with you, adapting to your improving fitness levels.

Recap and Moving Forward

Congratulations on embracing the power of fitness tracking with wearables! You've taken the first step toward a more active and health-conscious lifestyle. Remember, it's not just about the data, it's about the positive impact these digital tools can have on your well-being.

Key Takeaways:

- Wearables are your fitness companions, offering real-time tracking and feedback.
- Setting and achieving fitness goals becomes a dynamic and rewarding journey with the help of wearables.

Ready for the next stage? In the next Chapter, we'll explore how AI coaches can elevate your fitness game to new heights. Have you experienced the motivation of hitting a fitness goal with your wearable? Share your stories in the comments below and inspire others on their wellness journey!

Personalized Workouts with AI Coaches

Welcome to the dynamic duo of your digital fitness journey, AI Coaches and mobile apps. In this chapter, we'll explore how artificial intelligence becomes your virtual fitness trainer, tailoring workouts to your needs, and how mobile apps seamlessly integrate to bring exercise programs right to your fingertips.

Personalized Workouts with AI Coaches

Your AI Fitness Ally

Meet your new workout partner, your AI Coach. This digital companion takes personalization to the next level, crafting fitness routines based on your goals, preferences, and even your body's responses to previous exercises. It's like having a personal trainer who knows you inside out.

Getting Started:
1. Profile Personalization: Input your fitness goals, preferred exercise types, and any restrictions or considerations into your AI Coach app.

2. Interactive Assessments: Many AI Coaches conduct initial assessments to understand your fitness level. Be honest, and let the AI get to know you.

3. Real-Time Adjustments: As you progress through workouts, your AI Coach adapts, ensuring each session remains challenging and effective.

The Power of Adaptive Learning

One of the magical aspects of AI Coaches is their ability to learn and evolve with you. The more you engage, the better they understand your strengths, weaknesses, and preferences. This adaptive learning ensures your workouts are not just effective but enjoyable.

Integrating Mobile Apps for Exercise Programs

The Pocket Gym

Your smartphone is not just a communication device, it's a gateway to a world of exercise programs and fitness guidance. Mobile apps bring workouts to your schedule, allowing you to exercise anywhere, anytime.

Simple Steps:

1. Explore Fitness Apps: Browse app stores for apps aligned with your fitness goals. Whether you're into high-intensity training or prefer yoga, there's an app for you.

2. Trial and Select: Experiment with different apps to find the ones that resonate with you. Many apps offer trial periods or free versions.

3. Set a Routine: Incorporate your chosen app's exercise programs into your daily routine. Consistency is key to reaping the benefits.

Recap and Moving Forward

You've now unlocked the power of personalized workouts with AI Coaches and discovered the convenience of mobile apps for exercise programs. As you integrate these digital tools into your fitness routine, remember that the key is consistency and enjoyment.

Key Takeaways:

- AI Coaches create personalized workouts tailored to your goals and preferences.
- Mobile apps bring exercise programs to your fingertips, making fitness accessible anytime, anywhere.

Ready for the next step? In Chapter 3, we'll delve into the world of tracking nutrition with apps, ensuring your digital wellness journey covers all aspects of a healthy lifestyle. Share your experiences with AI Coach workouts or favorite fitness apps in the comments below—let's inspire each other to reach new fitness heights!

Chapter 3

Nutritional Optimization with Technology

Tracking Nutrition with Apps

Welcome to the heart of your digital wellness journey, the chapter where technology meets nutrition for a comprehensive approach to your well-being. In this section, we'll explore the transformative power of nutritional tracking apps, guiding you toward a healthier and more informed relationship with food.

Tracking Nutrition with Apps

Your Digital Food Diary
Imagine having a personal nutrition assistant in your pocket, helping you make informed choices about what goes on your plate. That's the magic of nutritional tracking apps. These apps not only log your meals but also provide insights into your dietary habits, ensuring you're nourishing your body effectively.

Getting Started:
1. **Choose Your App:** Explore the myriad of nutrition-tracking apps available. Opt for one that aligns with your goals, whether it's weight loss, muscle gain, or overall well-being.
2. **Input Your Meals:** Use the app to log what you eat throughout the day. Most apps have extensive databases, making it easy to find and log food items.
3. **Set Nutritional Goals:** Define your nutritional objectives within the app. Whether it's tracking calorie intake, monitoring macronutrients, or increasing water consumption, your app can help you stay on track.

The Insightful Journey

One of the greatest benefits of nutritional tracking apps is the insight they provide into your eating habits. From calorie counts to nutrient breakdowns, these apps empower you to make conscious choices, fostering a healthier and more balanced diet.

Maximizing Nutrition for Wellness

Setting and Achieving Dietary Goals

Nutritional tracking apps are not just about recording what you eat, they're about setting and achieving dietary goals. Whether you're aiming for weight management, improving specific nutrient intake, or adopting a new eating pattern, these apps guide you toward success.

Simple Steps:
1. Define Your Objectives: Clearly outline your dietary goals. Whether it's reducing sugar intake or increasing fiber, your app can help you create a roadmap.
2. Regular Check-Ins: Use the app consistently to monitor your progress. Celebrate achievements, no matter how small, and adjust your goals as needed.
3. Explore Recipe Suggestions: Many apps offer recipe ideas based on your dietary preferences. Expand your culinary horizons while staying aligned with your nutritional goals.

Recap and Moving Forward
You've now uncovered the potential of tracking nutrition with apps, a key element in your digital wellness arsenal. As you continue this journey, remember that understanding and optimizing your nutrition is a vital component of your overall health and fitness.

Key Takeaways:
- Nutritional tracking apps serve as your digital food diary, providing insights into your eating habits.

- Set and achieve dietary goals with the help of these apps, fostering a healthier relationship with food.

Ready for the next step? In the next chapter, we'll explore the world of AI-assisted meal planning, ensuring your nutritional journey is not just tracked but also optimized. Share your experiences with nutritional tracking apps in the comments below, let's inspire each other on the path to better nutrition!**

AI-Assisted Meal Planning

Welcome to the cutting edge of your digital wellness expedition, where artificial intelligence meets your dinner plate. In this chapter, we'll explore the wonders of AI-assisted meal planning, ensuring that your nutritional journey is not just tracked but optimized. Additionally, we'll delve into the fascinating realm of wearables and how they provide invaluable insights into your dietary habits.

AI-Assisted Meal Planning

Your Culinary Genius

Imagine having a virtual chef who understands your nutritional needs, preferences, and goals. AI-assisted meal planning does just that, it transforms the process of deciding what to eat into a personalized, efficient, and health-focused experience.

Getting Started:

1. Connect Your Data: Ensure that your nutritional tracking app is synced with your AI-assisted meal planning tool. This connection allows the AI to access real-time information about your dietary habits.

2. Set Dietary Preferences: Communicate your culinary preferences, dietary restrictions, and goals to the AI. Whether you're vegetarian, aiming for weight loss, or optimizing for a specific nutrient, the AI can tailor recommendations accordingly.

3. Explore and Confirm Suggestions: Let the AI generate meal suggestions based on your profile. Review the options, make adjustments as needed, and confirm your personalized meal plan.

The Smart Culinary Experience

AI-assisted meal planning is more than just a list of recipes. It's a dynamic process that adapts to your evolving nutritional needs. The AI considers factors such as your fitness goals, dietary restrictions, and even seasonal ingredients to create a truly personalized and sustainable eating plan.

Leveraging Wearables for Dietary Insights

Your Wearable Nutrition Tracker

Wearables are not limited to counting steps, they can also provide valuable insights into your dietary habits. These devices, equipped with advanced sensors, can monitor aspects like chewing patterns, eating pace, and even stress levels, offering a comprehensive view of your relationship with food.

Simple Steps:

1. Enable Nutrition Tracking: Ensure that your wearable nutrition tracking feature is activated. This might involve adjusting settings or installing specific apps.

2. Wear Consistently: To obtain accurate dietary insights, wear your device consistently during meals. This ensures comprehensive data collection.

3. Review Dietary Feedback: Many wearables provide feedback on your eating habits. Use this information to make conscious choices and adjust your meal patterns if necessary.

Recap and Moving Forward

Congratulations on embracing the power of AI-assisted meal planning and leveraging wearables for dietary insights. As you continue this nutritional journey, remember that personalized meal planning goes beyond just meeting your dietary needs—it's about enhancing your overall well-being.

Key Takeaways:

- AI-assisted meal planning personalizes your culinary experience based on your preferences and nutritional goals.
- Wearables provide valuable insights into your eating habits, promoting mindfulness and informed dietary choices.

*Ready for the next adventure? In Chapter 4, we'll explore the nuances of monitoring and improving your sleep with wearables, ensuring a holistic approach to your digital wellness. Have you tried an AI-assisted meal planning app or used your wearable for nutritional insights? Share your experiences in the comments below, let's learn from each other on the journey to optimal well-being!

Chapter 4

Revolutionizing Sleep Health

Monitoring Sleep Patterns with Wearables

Welcome to the realm of rejuvenation, Chapter 4, where we explore the transformative power of wearables in revolutionizing sleep health. In this section, we'll delve into the magic of monitoring sleep patterns with wearables, unlocking the secrets to a more restful and revitalizing night's sleep.

Monitoring Sleep Patterns with Wearables

Your Personal Sleep Scientist
Imagine having a sleep scientist right on your wrist, providing insights into the quality and duration of your nightly rest. Wearables equipped with advanced sleep tracking features do just that, they offer a window into your sleep patterns, helping you understand and optimize your sleep health.

Getting Started:

1. Activate Sleep Tracking: Ensure that your wearable sleep tracking feature is enabled. This might involve adjusting settings or installing specific apps.

2. Wear Comfortably: Wear your device consistently during the night. Most wearables are designed to be comfortable, allowing you to forget you're wearing them as they work diligently to monitor your sleep.

3. Review Sleep Data: In the morning, sync your wearable with its accompanying app to review detailed insights into your sleep patterns. Look for information on the duration of each sleep stage, interruptions, and overall sleep quality.

The Wisdom of Wearable Sleep Data

Sleep-tracking wearables go beyond simply recording the hours you spend in bed. They provide a comprehensive overview of your sleep cycles, including light sleep, deep sleep, and REM (rapid eye movement) sleep. Armed with this knowledge, you can make informed decisions to improve the quality of your rest.

Enhancing Sleep Hygiene

Making Informed Sleep Decisions

Monitoring sleep patterns isn't just about gathering data, it's about making informed decisions to enhance your sleep hygiene. Wearables provide actionable insights, suggesting adjustments to your bedtime routine, sleep environment, and overall lifestyle to promote better sleep.

Simple Steps:
1. Review Sleep Trends: Identify patterns in your sleep data, such as consistent bedtime and wake-up times.
2. Adjust Bedtime Routine: Based on your sleep data, consider incorporating relaxation techniques or minimizing screen time before bed.
3. Optimize Sleep Environment: Use wearables to assess the impact of changes in your sleep environment, such as room temperature and lighting, on your sleep quality.

Recap and Moving Forward
Congratulations on stepping into the world of monitoring sleep patterns with wearables. As you continue this journey, remember that a good night's sleep is a cornerstone of overall well-being. By harnessing the insights provided by wearables, you're empowered to make informed choices for a more restful and rejuvenating sleep.

Key Takeaways:
- Wearables equipped with sleep tracking features offer insights into the duration and quality of your sleep.
- Analyzing sleep data empowers you to make informed decisions to enhance your sleep hygiene.

Ready for the next stage? we'll explore stress management and mental well-being with the aid of mobile apps. Have you tried monitoring your sleep patterns with a wearable? Share your experiences in the comments below, let's continue to learn and support each other on the journey to optimal sleep health!**

Sleep Improvement Apps and Techniques

Welcome to the chapter dedicated to the art of mastering sleep, Here, we'll delve into the realm of sleep improvement apps and techniques, exploring how artificial intelligence can be harnessed to enhance the quality of your nightly rest.

Crafting Your Ideal Sleep Routine

Sleep improvement is an art, and it begins with cultivating healthy sleep habits and incorporating effective techniques into your bedtime routine. Sleep improvement apps act as valuable companions, offering guidance, relaxation exercises, and personalized strategies to optimize your sleep.

Getting Started:

1. Explore Sleep Apps: Browse app stores for sleep improvement apps. Look for those that align with your needs, whether it's reducing stress, improving relaxation, or addressing specific sleep challenges.

2. Establish a Routine: Set a consistent bedtime routine with the help of your chosen sleep app. This might involve activities such as meditation, gentle stretching, or guided imagery.

3. Track Your Progress: Many sleep improvement apps allow you to monitor your sleep patterns and the effectiveness of your routine. Regularly review your sleep data to refine and enhance your approach.

Techniques for a Restful Night
In addition to apps, incorporating specific techniques into your pre-sleep ritual can significantly impact the quality of your sleep. Techniques like progressive muscle relaxation, deep breathing exercises, and mindfulness can help calm the mind and prepare the body for a restful night.

Using AI for Sleep Quality Enhancement

Your AI Sleep Companion

Artificial intelligence takes sleep enhancement to the next level by personalizing interventions based on your unique sleep patterns and challenges. AI-powered sleep apps analyze data gathered from wearables and user inputs to offer tailored suggestions, creating a dynamic and responsive sleep improvement experience.

Simple Steps:

1. Connect Your Wearable: Ensure your wearable device is synced with your AI-powered sleep app. This connection provides the app with real-time data on your sleep patterns.

2. Provide Feedback: Regularly update the app with information about your sleep quality, any disruptions, and the effectiveness of your sleep routine.

3. Review AI Recommendations: AI algorithms analyze your sleep data to generate personalized recommendations. These could include adjustments to your bedtime routine, environmental changes, or specific sleep-inducing techniques.

Recap and Moving Forward

Congratulations on exploring the world of sleep improvement apps, techniques, and the power of AI in enhancing sleep quality. As you continue to refine your sleep routine, remember that small changes can lead to significant improvements in the quality of your rest.

Key Takeaways:

- Sleep improvement apps offer guidance, relaxation exercises, and personalized strategies to optimize your sleep routine.
- AI-powered sleep apps use real-time data to provide tailored recommendations, enhancing the effectiveness of your sleep enhancement efforts.

Ready for the next chapter? In Chapter 6, we'll delve into the role of AI in preventative care and how technology can contribute to the early detection and monitoring of health issues. Have you tried a sleep improvement app or experienced the benefits of AI-enhanced sleep techniques? Share your insights in the comments below, let's continue supporting each other on the path to optimal sleep health!**

Chapter 5

Preventative Care in the Digital Age

Early Detection and Monitoring with Wearables

Welcome to the forefront of healthcare innovation, where we explore the transformative role of preventative care in the digital age. In this section, we'll delve into the power of wearables, demonstrating how these digital companions contribute to the early detection and monitoring of health issues, empowering you to take proactive control of your well-being.

Your Personal Health Sentinel
Wearables have evolved beyond simple activity trackers, they now serve as your vigilant health guardians. Equipped with an array of sensors, these devices monitor vital signs, detect anomalies, and provide real-time data, offering a proactive approach to health management.

Getting Started:

1. Choose a Comprehensive Wearable: Opt for a wearable that goes beyond basic fitness tracking. Look for features such as heart rate monitoring, ECG (electrocardiogram) capabilities, sleep tracking, and other health-focused functionalities.

2. Set Up Health Alerts: Configure your wearable to provide alerts for abnormal health readings. This might include irregular heartbeats, sudden changes in sleep patterns, or prolonged periods of inactivity.

3. Regularly Review Health Data: Establish a routine for reviewing the health data collected by your wearable. Many devices sync seamlessly with mobile apps, providing detailed insights into your vital signs over time.

The Proactive Health Journey

The true power of wearables lies in their ability to detect potential health issues early, allowing for timely intervention and preventative measures. By actively monitoring key health indicators, wearables become proactive partners in your health journey.

Proactive Health Management

Navigating Your Health Landscape

Wearables not only detect anomalies but also assist in the ongoing management of your health. They provide valuable insights into your overall well-being, empowering you to make informed decisions about your lifestyle, habits, and healthcare choices.

Simple Steps:

1. Utilize Health Trends: Many wearables track trends over time, highlighting areas of improvement or stability. Use this information to adjust your health goals and monitor the effectiveness of lifestyle changes.

2. Share Data with Healthcare Providers: When seeking medical advice, share the data collected by your wearable with your healthcare team. This collaboration enhances their understanding of your health and aids in more accurate diagnoses and personalized care.

3. Act on Insights: Pay attention to trends and changes in your health data. If you notice persistent anomalies, consult with your healthcare provider for further evaluation and guidance.

Recap and Moving Forward

Congratulations on unlocking the potential of wearables in preventative care. As you continue on this proactive health journey, remember that early detection and monitoring empower you to make informed decisions, enhancing your well-being and fostering a proactive approach to health.

Key Takeaways:
- Wearables serve as personal health sentinels, monitoring vital signs and detecting anomalies.
- Proactive health management involves regularly reviewing health data, acting on insights, and collaborating with healthcare providers.

Ready for the next chapter? we'll explore the role of AI in personalized fitness coaching, helping you achieve your health and wellness goals with tailored guidance. Have you experienced the benefits of wearables in early detection? Share your insights and stories in the comments below, let's continue to inspire and support each other on the path to optimal health!

Mobile Apps for Health Checkups

Welcome to the frontier of personalized health managemen. In this section, we'll explore the convenience of mobile apps for health checkups and the revolutionary role that artificial intelligence (AI) plays in preventing health issues. Get ready to harness the power of technology for proactive and personalized well-being.

Your Pocket Health Companion
Mobile apps have redefined the concept of health checkups, offering accessible and user-friendly tools for monitoring various aspects of your well-being. From tracking vitals to providing personalized health insights, these apps empower you to take an active role in managing your health.

Getting Started:
1. Explore Health Checkup Apps: Browse app stores for health checkup apps that align with your health goals. Look for features such as symptom tracking, medication reminders, and integration with wearables.
2. Input Comprehensive Health Data: Provide relevant information about your health history, current symptoms, and lifestyle habits. The

more accurate the input, the more tailored the app's recommendations.

3. Regularly Update Health Data: Keep your health data up-to-date. Many apps offer features to track changes in symptoms, medication adherence, and other health metrics over time.

The Convenience of Personalized Health Insights

Mobile health checkup apps provide more than just data, they offer personalized insights and recommendations based on your health profile. Whether it's flagging potential issues, suggesting lifestyle adjustments, or providing medication reminders, these apps are your virtual health assistants.

The Role of AI in Preventing Health Issues

Your AI Health Guardian

Artificial intelligence takes preventative care to new heights by analyzing vast amounts of health data to identify patterns, trends, and potential risk factors. AI-powered health apps become your proactive health guardians, offering personalized recommendations to prevent health issues before they escalate.

Simple Steps:

1. Connect Your Health Data: Many health apps integrate with wearables, providing a comprehensive dataset for AI analysis. Ensure seamless connectivity for accurate insights.

2. AI-Enhanced Monitoring: Allow AI algorithms to analyze your health data over time. These algorithms can identify subtle changes and patterns that may not be immediately apparent.

3. Receive Personalized Recommendations: Based on the AI analysis, receive personalized recommendations for lifestyle adjustments, preventive measures, and early interventions.

Recap and Moving Forward

Congratulations on embracing the convenience of mobile apps for health checkups and harnessing the power of AI in preventative care. As you continue on this proactive health journey, remember that the combination of mobile technology and artificial intelligence empowers you to take charge of your health in unprecedented ways.

Key Takeaways:
- Mobile health checkup apps provide personalized insights and recommendations based on your health data.
- AI plays a crucial role in preventative care, offering early detection and personalized interventions to prevent health issues.

Ready for the next chapter? we'll explore the integration of technology into mental well-being, including AI-driven solutions for stress management. Have you experienced the benefits of mobile health checkup apps or AI-driven preventative care? Share your insights and stories in the comments below—let's continue to inspire and support each other on the journey to optimal health!**

Chapter 6

Caring for Mental Wellbeing

Mental Health Tracking with Wearables

Welcome to the pivotal chapter dedicated to the often-overlooked realm of mental wellbeing. In this section, we'll explore the significance of mental health tracking with wearables, highlighting how these devices can serve as valuable companions in your journey toward mental wellness.

Your Wearable Wellness Advocate
Beyond step counts and heart rates, wearables are evolving to become comprehensive tools for monitoring mental health. Equipped with sensors and algorithms, these devices offer insights into stress levels, sleep quality, and overall emotional well-being, providing a holistic approach to self-care.

Getting Started:
1. Choose a Mental Health-Focused Wearable:
Opt for wearables that explicitly offer mental

health tracking features. Look for devices with heart rate variability monitoring, stress tracking, and sleep quality analysis.

2. Configure Mental Health Settings: Set up your wearable mental health features according to your preferences. This might involve adjusting stress level thresholds, activating mindfulness prompts, or customizing sleep-tracking settings.

3. Wear Consistently: For accurate mental health tracking, wear your device consistently, especially during moments of potential stress or when monitoring sleep patterns.

The Holistic Mental Wellness Journey

Mental health tracking with wearables goes beyond identifying stress, it offers a comprehensive view of your mental wellness journey. By analyzing patterns over time, these wearables provide actionable insights, helping you make informed decisions for improved mental health.

Nurturing Emotional Resilience

Proactive Stress Management

Mental health tracking with wearables empowers you to be proactive in managing stress. By receiving real-time alerts and insights into stress levels, you can implement coping strategies, whether it's taking a break, practicing mindfulness, or engaging in activities that bring joy.

Simple Steps:

1. Respond to Stress Alerts: Configure your wearable to provide alerts when stress levels rise. Take these prompts seriously and pause for a moment of self-reflection or relaxation.

2. Incorporate Mindfulness Practices: Many wearables offer guided breathing exercises or mindfulness prompts. Integrate these practices into your routine to build emotional resilience.

3. Review Stress Trends: Regularly review the trends in your stress data. Identify patterns and potential triggers, allowing you to make proactive lifestyle adjustments.

Recap and Moving Forward

Congratulations on recognizing the importance of mental well-being and leveraging the capabilities of wearables for mental health tracking. As you continue on this holistic journey, remember that small, consistent efforts can lead to significant improvements in your emotional resilience and overall mental health.

Key Takeaways:

- Wearables with mental health tracking features offer a holistic approach to emotional well-being.
- Proactive stress management, guided by insights from wearables, can significantly improve mental health.

Ready for the next chapter? we'll delve into the world of AI-driven solutions for stress management and mental wellness. Have you explored mental health tracking with wearables? Share your experiences and insights in the comments below, let's continue to support and inspire each other on the path to optimal mental well-being!

Mobile Apps for Stress Management

Welcome to the forefront of mental wellness innovation. In this section, we'll explore the dynamic intersection of mobile apps and artificial intelligence (AI), providing you with powerful tools for stress management and comprehensive mental wellness support.

Your Portable Stress Relief Companion
Mobile apps dedicated to stress management offer a wealth of resources, from guided relaxation exercises to mood tracking features. Accessible at your fingertips, these apps are designed to help you navigate daily stressors and foster a healthier relationship with your mental well-being.

Getting Started:
1. Explore Stress Management Apps: Browse app stores for stress management apps tailored to your preferences. Look for features such as guided meditation, stress tracking, and personalized relaxation exercises.

2. Create a Personalized Routine: Incorporate stress management activities into your daily routine using the app. Whether it's a morning meditation or an evening wind-down session, consistency is key.

3. Track Your Stress Levels: Many apps allow you to monitor stress trends over time. Regularly check in on your stress levels and adjust your routine based on the insights provided.

The Empowerment of Self-Care

Mobile apps for stress management go beyond offering immediate relief—they empower you with the knowledge and tools to actively participate in your mental wellness journey. By integrating self-care into your routine, these apps foster long-term resilience and emotional well-being.

AI-Based Mental Wellness Support

Your AI Wellness Companion

Artificial intelligence adds a new dimension to mental wellness support by offering personalized and adaptive interventions. AI-driven mental wellness apps analyze your usage patterns, responses, and even physiological data to tailor recommendations that evolve with your unique needs.

Simple Steps:

1. Engage with AI Features: Explore and interact with the AI-driven features of your mental wellness app. This might include mood tracking, personalized recommendations, or conversational interfaces.

2. Provide Feedback: Many AI apps prompt you for feedback on the effectiveness of interventions. Share your experiences to fine-tune the app's suggestions.

3. Allow for Personalization: AI adapts to your unique preferences and responses. Be open to the evolving nature of the app's recommendations as it refines its understanding of your mental wellness journey.

Recap and Moving Forward

Congratulations on exploring the world of mobile apps for stress management and embracing AI-based mental wellness support. As you continue on this path, remember that the integration of technology can be a powerful ally in fostering a resilient and balanced mental well-being.

Key Takeaways:
- Mobile apps for stress management offer accessible tools for daily self-care and emotional well-being.
- AI-driven mental wellness support provides personalized interventions that adapt to your unique needs.

Ready for the next chapter? In Chapter 8, we'll delve into the importance of preventative mental health measures and the role of technology in early intervention. Share your experiences with stress management apps and AI-driven mental wellness support in the comments below, let's continue to learn and support each other on the journey to optimal mental health!

Chapter 7

Integration and Synergy of Digital Health Tools

Creating a Holistic Health Ecosystem

Welcome to a pivotal chapter where we explore the seamless integration and synergy of various digital health tools, forging the path toward a holistic health ecosystem. In this section, we'll dive into the interconnected world of health technology, where wearables, apps, and AI converge to create a comprehensive and personalized approach to well-being.

The Interconnected Web of Digital Wellness
Imagine a health journey where your wearable seamlessly communicates with your health app, and AI algorithms provide personalized insights, all working in harmony to support your holistic well-being. The integration and synergy of digital health tools transform fragmented data into a cohesive narrative of your health.

Getting Started:

1. Connect Your Devices: Ensure that your wearables, health-tracking apps, and AI-driven tools are interconnected. This might involve syncing data, enabling integrations, or using platforms that support cross-device compatibility.

2. Set Unified Health Goals: Establish overarching health goals that align with various aspects of your well-being, from physical fitness to mental health. Your holistic health ecosystem should work cohesively to address these objectives.

3. Regularly Review Comprehensive Data: Dive into the aggregated data from your interconnected tools regularly. Look for patterns, correlations, and areas of improvement that can inform your health decisions.

The Power of Unified Insights

The integration of digital health tools provides you with unified insights that extend beyond isolated metrics. By analyzing data collaboratively, your health ecosystem becomes a dynamic source of information, guiding you toward informed decisions for improved health.

Navigating a Personalized Health Journey

Tailored Recommendations for Well-Being
The synergy of digital health tools goes beyond data integration, it enables the delivery of personalized recommendations. AI algorithms, informed by a comprehensive view of your health, can offer tailored insights, interventions, and guidance for a truly individualized health journey.

Simple Steps:
1. Engage with AI Features: Actively participate in the AI-driven features of your health ecosystem. This might involve answering prompts, providing feedback, or following personalized recommendations.

2. Adjust Settings for Personalization: Customize the settings of your digital health tools to enhance personalization. This could include refining stress level thresholds, adjusting fitness targets, or fine-tuning nutrition goals.

3. Celebrate Milestones and Adjust Goals: As you progress on your health journey, celebrate achievements and adjust goals. Your holistic health ecosystem should evolve with you, accommodating changes in your lifestyle, preferences, and well-being.

Recap and Moving Forward

Congratulations on establishing and nurturing your holistic health ecosystem, where digital tools synergize to create a personalized and comprehensive approach to well-being. As you continue on this interconnected journey, remember that the power of your health ecosystem lies in its ability to adapt and evolve with you.

Key Takeaways:
- The integration of digital health tools creates a unified and comprehensive view of your well-being.
- A holistic health ecosystem offers personalized insights and recommendations, fostering a tailored approach to individual health.

Ready for the next chapter? we'll explore the future of digital health and the ongoing evolution of technology in shaping our well-being. Share your experiences with creating a holistic health ecosystem in the comments below, let's continue to inspire and support each other on the journey to optimal health!

Interconnectedness of Wearables, Apps, and AI

Welcome to the culmination of our exploration, the interconnected landscape where wearables, apps, and artificial intelligence (AI) converge to maximize health benefits. In Chapter 8, we delve into the synergistic potential of these digital tools, revealing how their seamless integration elevates well-being to new heights.

The Symphony of Digital Well-Being
Imagine your wearable acting as the rhythm section, your health app playing the melody, and AI orchestrating the harmonies, the result is a symphony of interconnected digital tools working in concert to enhance your health. This chapter explores how the integration of wearables, apps, and AI creates a holistic and personalized approach to well-being.

Getting Started:
1. Establish Unified Health Goals: Define comprehensive health goals that encompass physical fitness, mental well-being, and preventive care. These goals will guide the integration and collaboration of your digital tools.

2. Ensure Seamless Connectivity: Confirm that your wearables and apps seamlessly connect and share data. Many platforms offer integration settings that enhance the interoperability of these tools.

3. Leverage AI for Unified Insights: Explore AI-driven features that consolidate data from wearables and apps. This AI integration can provide deeper insights, predictive analytics, and personalized recommendations for your health journey.

The Holistic Health Advantage

Integration transforms isolated data points into a holistic narrative of your health. By fostering communication and collaboration among wearables, apps, and AI, you gain a comprehensive understanding of your well-being, enabling targeted interventions and proactive health management.

Nurturing Personalized Health Journeys

The interconnectedness of digital tools enables a tailored approach to health management. By utilizing AI algorithms, wearables, and apps can deliver personalized guidance, adapt to your evolving needs, and empower you to navigate a health journey that is uniquely yours.

Simple Steps:

1. Engage with Personalization Features: Actively participate in the personalization features of your digital tools. Provide feedback, answer prompts, and adjust settings to refine the tailored guidance.

2. Review Unified Health Data: Regularly review the insights generated by the integration of wearables, apps, and AI. Identify patterns, trends, and areas for improvement that inform your personalized health goals.

3. Celebrate Milestones and Adjust Strategies: Acknowledge achievements and adjust strategies based on the evolving feedback from your digital health ecosystem. This dynamic approach ensures continuous adaptation to your well-being needs.

Recap and Moving Forward

Congratulations on embracing the interconnected world of wearables, apps, and AI to maximize health benefits. As you reflect on this journey, remember that the true power lies in the ongoing collaboration of these tools, continually adapting to nurture your well-being.

Key Takeaways:
- The integration of wearables, apps, and AI creates a symphony of digital well-being.
- A holistic and personalized health approach is realized through the interconnectedness of these digital tools.

Ready for the next chapter? In our concluding chapter, we'll explore the future of digital health, anticipating the innovations and advancements that will shape the ongoing evolution of well-being. Share your thoughts on the interconnectedness of digital tools in the comments below, let's continue to inspire and support each other on the journey to optimal health!**

Chapter 8

Challenges and Ethical Considerations

Addressing Privacy Concerns

Welcome to the final chapter of our exploration, a critical examination of challenges and ethical considerations surrounding the integration of digital health tools. In Chapter 8, we'll navigate the complex terrain of privacy concerns, ethical use of health data, and strategies to overcome challenges in the widespread adoption of digital wellness.

Safeguarding Your Digital Health Journey
The integration of wearables, apps, and AI raises legitimate concerns about the privacy and security of health data. As users entrust these tools with sensitive information, it's essential to implement robust measures to protect privacy.

Protective Measures:
1. Review Privacy Settings: Regularly review and adjust the privacy settings of your digital

health tools. Familiarize yourself with the options available for controlling data sharing, visibility, and third-party access.

2. Understand Data Ownership: Clarify the ownership of your health data. Ensure that your chosen tools have transparent policies regarding who owns the data and how it can be used.

3. Choose Secure Platforms: Prioritize tools and platforms with a strong reputation for data security. Research and select options that implement encryption, secure storage practices, and stringent access controls.

Ethical Use of Health Data

The ethical use of health data is paramount in the digital wellness landscape. As users contribute valuable insights into their well-being, developers, providers, and policymakers must uphold ethical standards and respect user autonomy.

Ethical Guidelines:

1. Informed Consent: Prioritize platforms that prioritize informed consent. Users should be fully aware of how their health data will be used, shared, and analyzed, allowing for an informed decision.

2. Anonymization and Aggregation: Advocate for platforms that employ anonymization and aggregation techniques. This ensures that individual health data is transformed into formats that protect identity while still contributing to valuable insights.

3. User Control: Support platforms that grant users control over their health data. This includes the ability to delete data, restrict access, and determine sharing preferences.

Overcoming Challenges in Digital Wellness Adoption

Despite the tremendous potential of digital wellness tools, challenges persist in achieving widespread adoption. Identifying and addressing these barriers is essential for maximizing the positive impact of these technologies on public health.

Strategic Approaches:

1. Education and Awareness: Promote education and awareness campaigns to inform the public about the benefits and safety measures associated with digital wellness tools. Addressing misconceptions is key to fostering trust.

2. Interoperability Standards: Advocate for the development and adoption of interoperability standards. Seamless integration between different digital health tools encourages a unified and user-friendly experience.

3. Affordability and Accessibility: Work towards making digital wellness tools more affordable and accessible. This includes exploring partnerships, subsidies, and initiatives to ensure that these technologies are within reach for diverse populations.

Recap and Moving Forward

As we conclude our journey, it's crucial to acknowledge and address the challenges and ethical considerations surrounding the integration of digital health tools. By actively engaging in privacy protection, promoting ethical use of health data, and overcoming adoption barriers, we pave the way for a future where digital wellness is inclusive, secure, and empowering for all.

Key Takeaways:

- Privacy concerns demand continuous vigilance through user-controlled settings and informed consent.
- The ethical use of health data requires transparent practices, anonymization, and respect for user autonomy.
- Overcoming challenges in adoption involves education, interoperability standards, and efforts to enhance affordability and accessibility.

Thank you for joining us on this exploration of the transformative landscape of digital wellness. As we look to the future, may our collective efforts ensure that these technologies contribute positively to the health and well-being of individuals and communities. Feel free to share your thoughts on challenges and ethical considerations in the digital wellness space in the comments below, let's continue the conversation and support one another on the path to optimal health!

Chapter 9

Future Trends in Digital Wellness

Emerging Technologies in Health

Welcome to the visionary realm of Chapter 9, where we explore the exciting frontiers of digital wellness. In this section, we'll gaze into the future, anticipating the emergence of groundbreaking technologies in health, envisioning the evolution of wearables and apps, and contemplating the transformative journey of artificial intelligence (AI) in healthcare.

Pioneering the Next Wave of Well-Being

The future promises an array of innovative technologies that will redefine how we approach health and wellness. From advanced diagnostics to personalized treatments, emerging technologies are poised to revolutionize the landscape of digital health.

Anticipated Trends:

1. Genomic Medicine: The decoding of the human genome opens the door to personalized treatments based on individual genetic makeup.

2. Telehealth Advancements: The integration of virtual reality (VR) and augmented reality (AR) will enhance the capabilities of telehealth, providing immersive and interactive healthcare experiences.

3. Nanotechnology in Healthcare: Nanoscale technologies hold the potential for precise drug delivery, diagnostics, and monitoring at a cellular level.

Anticipated Developments in Wearables and Apps

The evolution of wearables and apps will not only continue but will accelerate, offering users increasingly sophisticated and personalized health experiences. From advanced sensing capabilities to seamless integration with daily life, these tools are set to redefine how we engage with our well-being.

Envisioned Advancements:

1. Biosensors for Comprehensive Monitoring: Wearables equipped with advanced biosensors will provide real-time monitoring of a wide range of health metrics, offering a comprehensive view of well-being.

2. Integration with Smart Environments: Wearables and apps will seamlessly integrate with smart homes and cities, creating an interconnected ecosystem that supports health-conscious living.

3. Emphasis on Mental Health Features: Mental health-focused features, including advanced stress detection and personalized mindfulness programs, will become standard in wearables and apps.

The Evolution of AI in Healthcare

The journey of AI in healthcare is poised to become even more transformative, with advancements ranging from diagnostic accuracy to personalized treatment recommendations. The evolving role of AI promises to empower individuals and healthcare professionals alike.

Envisaged Developments:

1. AI-Assisted Diagnostics: AI algorithms will continue to enhance diagnostic accuracy, enabling early detection of diseases and improving overall healthcare outcomes.

2. Personalized Treatment Plans: AI-driven insights, considering individual health data and genetic information, will contribute to the creation of highly personalized treatment plans.

3. Conversational AI in Mental Health Support: AI-powered chatbots and virtual assistants will play an increasingly prominent role in providing mental health support, and offering personalized interventions and resources.

Recap and Looking Ahead

As we peer into the future of digital wellness, the possibilities are exhilarating. Emerging technologies, advancements in wearables and apps, and the continued evolution of AI in healthcare collectively chart a course toward a future where health is not only monitored but actively enhanced through personalized, innovative, and interconnected digital solutions.

Key Takeaways:
- Emerging technologies include genomic medicine, advanced telehealth, and nanotechnology.
- Anticipated developments in wearables and apps encompass biosensors, smart environment integration, and a heightened focus on mental health features.
- The evolution of AI in healthcare promises enhanced diagnostics, personalized treatment plans, and conversational AI in mental health support.

Exciting times lie ahead in the digital wellness landscape. What are your thoughts on these future trends? Share your insights and aspirations in the comments below, let's continue to inspire and support each other on the journey to a future of optimal health and well-being!

Conclusion

As we draw the final curtain on our exploration of "Transform Your Health with Digital Wellness," the tapestry of insights, possibilities, and transformative technologies unfolds before us. This journey through the realms of wearables, mobile apps, AI, and emerging health technologies has been nothing short of exhilarating.

In our pursuit of optimal health, we embarked on a voyage that transcended traditional boundaries. From the foundations of digital wellness to the interconnected symphony of wearables, apps, and AI, we've witnessed the evolution of personal well-being in the digital age. Our exploration touched upon personalized fitness, nutrition, sleep, preventative care, mental health, and the seamless integration of digital health tools to create holistic ecosystems.

As we gaze into the future, the horizon is adorned with promising trends, genomic medicine, telehealth advancements, biosensors, smart environments, and the ever-evolving intelligence of AI in healthcare. The digital wellness landscape is poised for a paradigm shift, promising not just monitoring but active enhancement of our health through innovative, personalized, and interconnected solutions.

Yet, with the promise of progress comes the responsibility to address challenges and ethical considerations. Safeguarding privacy, ensuring the ethical use of health data, and overcoming barriers to adoption are vital endeavors to cultivate trust and inclusivity in the digital wellness revolution.

In the grand tapestry of digital wellness, each chapter, concept, and insight has contributed to a narrative of empowerment, enlightenment, and inspiration. Whether you're just beginning your digital wellness journey or you're a seasoned navigator, the pages of this book are an invitation, a call to action to leverage the power of technology for transformative well-being.

As we conclude this chapter of our exploration, let's carry forward the lessons learned, the possibilities envisioned, and the camaraderie fostered. The future of digital wellness is a collective endeavor, one where individuals, communities, and technology converge to create a healthier, more connected world.

Thank you for joining us on this odyssey. May your digital wellness journey be filled with empowerment, discovery, and the realization of your healthiest, most vibrant self.

Here's to the future, a future where digital wellness is not just a concept but a living reality, shaping the well-being of generations to come. Safe travels on your continued journey to transform your health with digital wellness.